Navigating Nausea

A guide to managing pregnancy sickness

By

Erwin Torp

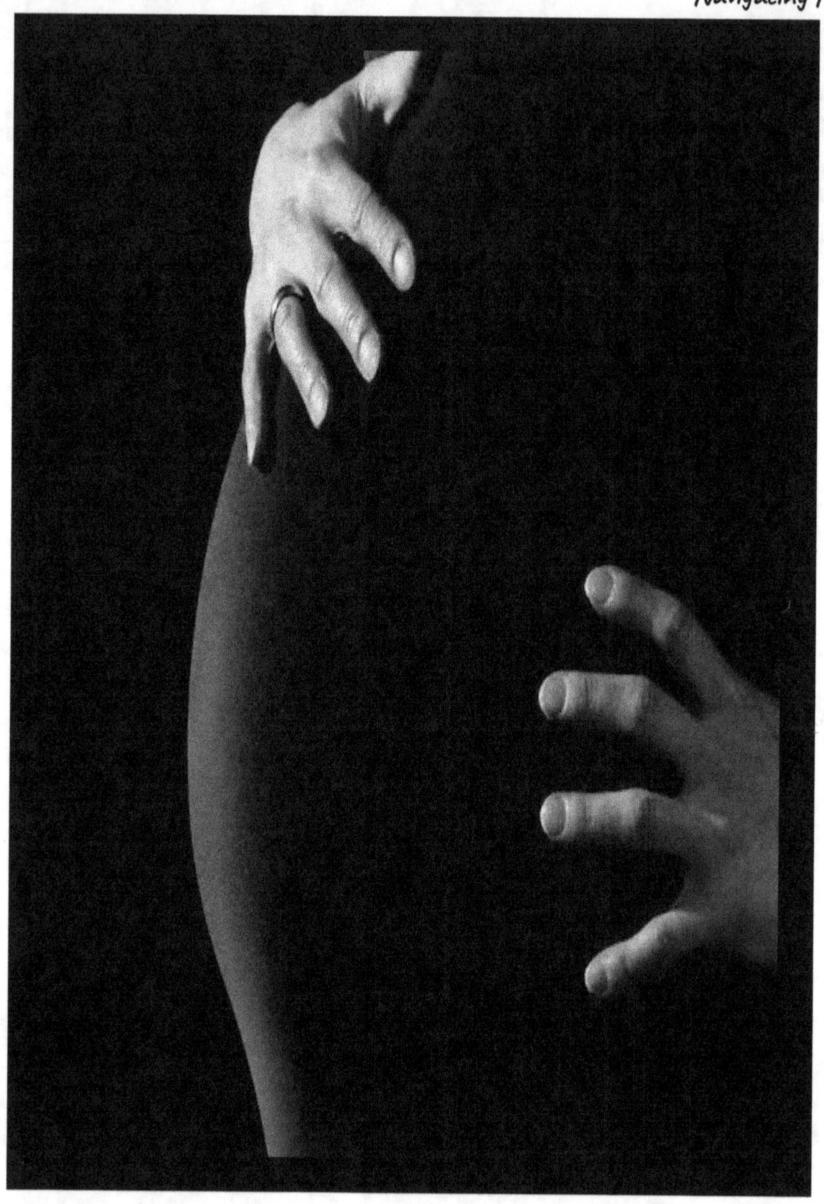

Table of Contents

Introduction

Starting the amazing journey of parenthood is a happy occasion for getting pregnant.

A woman's life is full of excitement and joy during her pregnancy.

Pregnancy sickness is one of the unanticipated difficulties that it may present.

Morning sickness, a common condition that many pregnant women experience is also known as pregnancy sickness.

It is typified by symptoms that can happen at any time of day, including fatigue, nausea, and vomiting.

Despite its name, morning sickness can strike some women and last all day.

In this book, we will examine pregnancy sickness's causes, signs, and possible remedies.

We will talk about how this condition develops and the physiological changes that take place during pregnancy.

We will also explore the various theories regarding the origins of pregnancy sickness and the current state of research on this phenomenon.

We will also offer helpful suggestions and guidance for handling pregnancy sickness.

We will look at a variety of treatment options that can help reduce symptoms and help expectant moms cope better during this time, from dietary adjustments to alternative therapies.

Furthermore, we will discuss the psychological and emotional effects of pregnancy sickness.

A woman's mental health may suffer when she has to deal with persistent nausea and vomiting.

We will talk about coping mechanisms for these difficulties.

Chapter 1

Understanding Pregnancy Sickness

Pregnant women frequently experience morning sickness, also referred to as pregnancy sickness.

It usually occurs during the first trimester, but for some women, it can last throughout the pregnancy.

It is characterized by feelings of nausea and occasionally vomiting.

Although the precise cause of pregnancy sickness remains unknown, it is thought that hormonal fluctuations, specifically elevated levels of estrogen and human chorionic gonadotropin (hCG), play a role in these symptoms.

The Intensity and duration of pregnancy sickness symptoms can differ.

Some women might feel a little queasy, while others might throw up more frequently and with greater intensity.

Pregnancy and pregnancy can also differ in the frequency and intensity of symptoms.

Although it usually strikes first thing in the morning when you wake up, morning sickness can last all day.

Some triggers, like particular foods or smells, can make the symptoms worse.

Pregnancy sickness can be upsetting and uncomfortable, but it is generally accepted as a normal aspect of the process and does not endanger the unborn child.

Morning sickness is not limited to the morning; it can strike at any time of day.

Although the symptoms usually go away on their own by the second trimester, they occasionally continue into the third trimester of pregnancy.

More severe pregnancy symptoms include hyperemesis gravidarum.

As the pregnancy goes on, the symptoms usually go away by the second trimester.
Some women, however, might endure mild symptoms for the duration of their pregnancy.

The expectant mother and her unborn child must recognize and treat pregnancy sickness.

If the symptoms are severe, persistent, or interfere with day-to-day functioning, it is advised to see a healthcare professional.

They can offer direction, encouragement, and, if required, medication prescriptions to treat symptoms.

Pregnancy sickness can be physically and psychologically taxing, so it's also critical to look after one's emotional health during this time.

To help you deal with the difficulties of pregnancy sickness, you can join pregnancy support groups or ask loved ones for assistance.

Remember that even though I make an effort to give accurate and current information, there's a chance that my answers don't always correspond with the most recent findings or recommendations from medical professionals.

For more detailed advice and direction on handling pregnancy sickness, it is therefore always advisable to speak with a healthcare provider.

Pregnancy-related illnesses' prevalence

The frequency of morning sickness, or pregnancy sickness, varies greatly depending on the population being studied and the criteria employed to describe the illness.

Still, estimates place the number of pregnant women experiencing some form of pregnancy sickness between 50 and 80 percent.

Individual differences also exist in the duration and intensity of symptoms.

While the majority of women only have mild symptoms like nausea and queasiness, some may have more severe symptoms that significantly impair their quality of life and ability to go about their daily activities.

It's crucial to remember that, despite the term "morning sickness" being widely used, this illness can strike at any time of day and, in some cases, persist the whole pregnancy.

Pregnancy symptoms

Pregnancy sickness, commonly referred to as morning sickness, often manifests as the following symptoms:

1. Nausea: Experiencing a strong feeling of nausea or the desire to throw up.
Secondly, vomiting is the involuntary, active evacuation of stomach contents.

2. Fatigue: Being extremely exhausted and lacking in vitality.

3. Loss of appetite: Feeling full after eating or having a diminished desire to eat.

4. Smell sensitivity: Experiencing

heightened sensitivity to specific scents, which may cause queasy feelings.

5. Dizziness: Feeling faint or lightheaded,

particularly after standing up too quickly.

6. Sensitive or tender breasts:

Feeling pain or discomfort around the breasts.

7. Urinating more frequently than usual: The need to urinate more

frequently.

8. mood swings: Feeling agitated,

sensitive to emotions more intensely, or both.

Additional signs of pregnancy symptoms include:

1. Food cravings: Cravings for specific foods, particularly those high in calcium and energy, like milk and other dairy products, are common during pregnancy.

You might also experience an abrupt dislike for meals that you used to enjoy.

Even strange tastes in non-food items like paper or soil can develop in some women.

Called "pica," this could be a sign of a nutrient shortage. If this persists, please consult your GP or midwife.

2. Back pain: More than 1 in 3 women experience back pain during pregnancy.

This typically results from changing posture brought on by the growing pregnancy and ligament loosening.

Wearing flat-heeled shoes, sitting in back-supporting chairs, avoiding heavy lifting, and engaging in mild

exercise can all help lessen back pain during pregnancy.

Back pain during pregnancy can be lessened by working out in the water.

Physiotherapy and acupuncture may also be beneficial.

3. Constipation: describes hard, infrequent bowel movements that are challenging to pass.

Pregnancy hormones can slow down your digestive system, or the pressure of your expanding uterus on your rectum can be the cause of this common pregnancy ailment.

It is recommended that you:

• Drink lots of water each day if you become constipated during pregnancy.

• Eat more high-fiber foods, such as wheat, bran,and fresh fruit and vegetables.

• Engage in mild, low-impact physical activities like yoga, walking, or swimming.

4. Migraine: During pregnancy, especially in the second half, get in touch with your doctor or midwife if you experience a headache that is not improved by paracetamol (like Panadol).

A chronic headache may be a sign of preeclampsia, a disorder that affects the kidneys and can raise blood pressure and reduce blood flow to the baby.

5. Indigestion and heartburn:

Acid from the stomach enters the esophagus and causes pain and discomfort, which is known as reflux or heartburn.

Pregnancy increases the risk of indigestion because of the expanding uterus's pressure on the abdominal organs and progesterone's ability to relax the muscle that separates the esophagus and stomach.

If you are experiencing heartburn, reflux, or indigestion.

It is advised that you:

• Eat smaller, more frequent meals if you are suffering from heartburn, reflux, or indigestion.

• Steer clear of food right before bed.

• Raise your head by using additional pillows while you sleep.

• Dress in baggy apparel.

• Steer clear of anything that exacerbates your symptoms, such as fatty meals (like fried foods, fatty meats, and pastries), spicy meals (like curry and chili), alcohol, and caffeine (like tea, coffee, and cola).

• Before taking an antacid, speak with your doctor.

5. Itchy skin: Please see your doctor if these methods are ineffective for your symptoms.

They might recommend a medication that will safely lower your acid secretion.

Though uncommon during pregnancy, widespread body itching can be extremely upsetting and

interfere with sleep and the enjoyment of the pregnancy.

Although eczema and dry skin are the most frequent causes, itching can occasionally have no apparent explanation.

A blood test can be performed to check for serious liver disease, which is a possible cause of itchy palms and soles of the feet in rare instances.

The body's reaction to the skin stretching later in pregnancy is thought to be the cause of an itchy rash. PUPPS is the name of this.

Moisturizers and antihistamines can be used to reduce itching.

Which antihistamines are safe to take while pregnant? Ask your doctor or midwife.

6. Leg cramps: An accumulation of acids results in the impacted muscles contracting uncontrollably.

Up to half of expectant mothers have them, usually at night.

During the second and third trimesters, leg cramps are more common.

The following actions are advised if you have leg cramps:

• Move around.

• To distribute the acid buildup, stretch and massage the affected muscle or muscles.

• Treat the afflicted muscle or muscles with a warm pack.

Consult your doctor or midwife about taking magnesium citrate or lactate in the morning and evening if cramps are causing you any discomfort.

7. Carpal tunnel syndrome: Which causes tingling and numbness in the hands, affects up to 60% of pregnant women.

Pregnancy-related increases in tissue fluids compress the median nerve, resulting in this condition.

The thumb's partial paralysis or loss of sensation may result from mild, sporadic, or severe carpal tunnel syndrome.

Soon after birth, symptoms typically go away on their own.

Tell your midwife or doctor if you have tingling or numbness in your hands.

Your doctor might suggest surgery or corticosteroid injections in extremely severe situations.

8. Virginal discharge: During

pregnancy, an increase in vaginal discharge is a common change.

If it is accompanied by pain, itchiness, an unpleasant smell, or discomfort when passing urine, an infection may be the cause.

Consult your GP for treatment.

9. Vaginitis: An uncomfortable ailment for

numerous women, vaginitis is an inflammation of the vagina. During pregnancy, it occurs more frequently.

Vaginal thrush, bacterial vaginosis, trichomonas, and Chlamydia are a few causes of vaginitis.

See your doctor for a diagnosis and course of action.

10. Varicose veins and leg edema (swelling): Pregnancy-related

varicose veins are highly prevalent because of

several factors, such as the larger veins being compressed by the growing uterus and the increased volume of blood flowing through the body.

In addition to causing pain, a heavy feeling in the legs, cramps (especially at night), and other strange sensations, this increased pressure on the veins can also cause edema or swelling of the legs.

The following actions are advised if you have varicose veins:

• Put on support stockings.

• Avoid standing for extended periods.

• Engage in regular, mild exercise (walking or swimming).

• When you can, raise your feet and lie down to rest.

• Give your legs a massage.

When you next visit your doctor or midwife, let them know.

Reasons why some women get pregnant and sick

The severity of morning sickness varies from woman to woman during pregnancy, and there is no single cause.

One of the most frequent causes during the first few weeks of pregnancy is elevated hormone levels. Another frequent reason for morning sickness is low blood sugar.

Morning sickness can be made worse by other things.

These consist of:

• Having triplets or twins.

• Being overly tired.

• Experiencing emotional stress.

• traveling frequently.

Throughout pregnancies, morning sickness can vary.

If you experienced severe morning sickness during one pregnancy, it might be very mild in subsequent pregnancies.

Potential side effects from morning sickness Appetite loss can be easily brought on by nausea and vomiting.

Pregnant women frequently fear for their unborn children's health.

Generally speaking, mild morning sickness is harmless.

If morning sickness persists after the first three to four months of pregnancy, pregnant women should consult their physician.

In addition, get assistance if you don't gain any weight while pregnant.

Most of the time, morning sickness is not severe enough to impair fetal development or growth.

Some pregnant women who experience nausea also lose weight and throw up a lot.

Hyperemesis gravidarum is the term for this condition.

It results in unintended weight loss and electrolyte imbalances.

This illness might eventually hurt your child if left untreated.

If you encounter any of the following symptoms, contact your doctor right away:

- Difficulty finishing meals
- Loss of two pounds or more in weight
- High fever
- Infrequent urination with tiny amounts of dark urine
- Fast heartbeat
- Severe nausea in the second trimester
- Blood in the vomit
- Frequent headaches
- Abdominal pain
- Spotting or bleeding

Strategies for Managing Morning Sickness

Your doctor may prescribe vitamins or nausea medication to help you remain hydrated and minimize nausea.

Your doctor might suggest any of the following drugs:

- **Metoclopramide (Reglan):** reduces nausea and vomiting and aids in the stomach's passage of food into the intestines.

- **Antacids:** they help stop acid reflux by absorbing stomach acid.

- **Antihistamines:** these relieve motion sickness and nausea.

- **Phenothiazine:** reduces extreme vomiting and nausea.

Do not use these medications by yourself without first talking to your doctor.

Some people have found relief from morning sickness with alternative remedies.

Before trying these, make sure you discuss them with your physician.

These therapies include:

- Extra vitamin B-6
- Pregnant women's vitamins
- Crackers with saltines
- Herbal medicine
- Psychotherapy
- Products made with ginger, like tea, drops, and ginger ale.

It is not to be confused with morning sickness, hyperemesis gravidarum, or other similar illnesses.

Hyperemesis gravidarum: what is it?

When severe, ongoing nausea and vomiting occur during pregnancy, it is known as hyperemesis gravidarum (HG).

Dehydration and weight loss may result from it. Another name for hyperemesis gravidarum is severe morning sickness.

Up to 80% of pregnant women report having morning sickness, which is incredibly common.

It is not as severe as hyperemesis gravidarum, and neither does it result in weight loss or dehydration.

You should still be able to avoid food and liquids for the majority of the day, even though morning sickness may occasionally cause nausea and vomiting.

After 12 weeks of pregnancy (the first trimester), it usually lessens or goes away entirely.

Vomiting occurs multiple times a day in patients with hyperemesis gravidarum.

Dehydration and weight loss may eventually result from this.
Morning sickness usually subsides before HG symptoms do.

If you become dehydrated, you may require hospital treatment, including IV fluids (fluids administered through a vein).

How frequent is gravidarum hyperemesis?

HG is rare. Less than 3% of pregnant women are affected.

What signs of hyperemesis gravidarum are present? Usually, starting around six weeks into your pregnancy, hyperemesis gravidarum happens in the first trimester.

Months, weeks, or even until delivery, symptoms may persist.

They might be crippling, keeping you from going about your everyday business.

What consequences might arise from gravidarum hyperemesis?

The majority of HG-related issues are brought on by malnourishment and a lack of fluids.

It is difficult for your body to absorb the necessary vitamins and nutrients when you throw up so much.

Complications like preterm birth or low birth weight could result from this.

Other side effects of excessive vomiting could include bleeding in your throat.

In what way is hyperemesis gravidarum identified?

Your doctor will conduct a physical examination, inquire about your symptoms, and review your medical history.

This involves determining whether you've lost too much weight by looking at your weight.

To check for dehydration, your doctor may prescribe blood and urine tests.

To check for signs of gastrointestinal disorders such as GTD, or if you are carrying more than one fetus, they might also use ultrasound.

What is the treatment for gravidarum hyperemesis?

The degree of your symptoms will determine how you are treated.

Make sure your pregnancy care provider is aware of all of your treatment options.

Possible treatments for very mild cases could be:

- **Lifestyle:** modifications such as donning an acupressure band or eating ginger chews and consuming ginger tea to relieve nausea.

- **Dietary adjustments:** Frequently eating small meals of dry, bland food every two hours can help reduce nausea and vomiting.

Good examples include crackers, toast, white potatoes, and rice.

Research indicates that eating a lot of fat during pregnancy may make you feel queasy.

Avoiding oily or spicy foods may be advised by your provider.

- **Anti-nausea drugs:** Several over-the-counter (OTC) drugs are effective against nausea.

Unisom doxylamine and pyridoxine (vitamin B6) are the most widely used.

If none of the above two remedies relieve your symptoms, your doctor might recommend an antihistamine such as diphenhydramine.

1. Prescription medication: Several prescription medications can reduce nausea and vomiting.

The first prescription your doctor will write for you will contain both B6 and doxylamine.

Stronger medicine might be required, though.

Promethazine and metoclopramide are the two most often prescribed drugs for nausea and vomiting.

Another medication that may be used to treat nausea and vomiting is ondansetron.

If you're unable to take some of these drugs orally, you can receive them via an IV, injection, or rectal suppository.

2. Intravenous fluids: An IV will be

inserted into your arm by your healthcare professional to give you nutrients and fluids.

Hospitalization may be necessary for this.

3. Tube feeding: A flexible tube inserted

into your stomach or nose by your healthcare
provider will provide you with nutrients.
You will typically receive treatment in a hospital.

4. Total parenteral intravenous

nutrition (TPN): In the most extreme

instances of hyperemesis gravidarum, an IV that

completely bypasses your digestive tract may be
necessary to provide nutrients.

This relieves pressure on your digestive system and
makes it self-healing.

Make sure you discuss with your healthcare provider the potential hazards of taking specific HG medications while pregnant.

When will the gravidarum hyperemesis end?

Yes.
You may not experience your symptoms after the first trimester.

It is also conceivable that your symptoms will last the whole time you are pregnant.

Many people report that the intensity of their symptoms decreases over time.

Thankfully, it almost always vanishes after delivery.

Is gravidarum hyperemesis preventable?

Avoiding hyperemesis gravidarum is not possible. Finding out if you are at risk is the best preparation you can make.

What consequences does hyperemesis gravidarum have on the developing fetus?

If your doctor is monitoring your pregnancy while you are undergoing treatment, HG frequently has little effect on the fetus.

Rarely, dehydration or excessive weight loss can cause your baby to be delivered smaller than normal.

When hyperemesis gravidarum happens, is pregnancy considered high-risk?

Your doctor will likely treat your pregnancy as high-risk.

This suggests that, to make sure there are no problems, your healthcare professional will monitor your pregnancy more closely.

In cases of hyperemesis gravidarum, what is the recommended treatment plan?

The best course of action for treating hyperemesis gravidarum is to speak with your provider.

The only person who can treat severe HG symptoms, like dehydration, is your provider.

Regarding further self-care steps you can take at home, follow your provider's recommendations.

For example, you may attempt the following:

• Consuming little meals every couple of hours.

• Eating boring food.

• Stay away from meals that make you fat.

• Using ginger, vitamin B6, and/or pressure-point wristbands to treat nausea.

• Avoid triggers, such as operating a vehicle.

When would it be best for me to visit my physician?

Pregnant women rarely have severe vomiting fits or have trouble putting food or beverages down.

It could be required to seek medical attention.

Immediately get in touch with your prenatal care provider if you encounter any of the following symptoms:

• severe nausea that keeps you from eating during the day.

• Have three or more episodes of vomiting per day for a few days.

• Lose a couple of inches.

• Experience dizziness, faintness, or confusion.

• Avoid urinating or urinating dimly. Busting myths regarding pregnancy that are widely held.

You may be experiencing a mental and physical rollercoaster as you embark on the amazing journey of parenting.

Pregnancy has many benefits, but it also has several disadvantages.

Morning sickness, or nausea and vomiting associated with pregnancy, is one of the most common.

Have you ever been there before?

If not, you might be curious about the potential effects nausea and vomiting may have on your fetus.

Our main objectives will be to debunk myths regarding this common pregnancy symptom and provide you with practical tips to help you through this stage.

Common Myths About Morning Sickness

1. Morning sickness only occurs in the morning:

This is one of the greatest myths regarding pregnancy sickness.

It is believed to only happen in the morning.
In actuality, these signs and symptoms can appear day or night.

While some expectant mothers may experience more intense symptoms in the morning, others may struggle with nausea and vomiting all day.

Though remembering that this variation is completely normal, it can still be confusing and frustrating.

It can be especially important for expectant mothers to comprehend this myth.

You might discover that your symptoms make it difficult for you to take care of your body and your developing child daily, which could leave you feeling inadequate or guilty.

You may feel nauseous, but don't worry—your baby will continue to be fed while you tend to your health.

If you need to take a break or seek assistance, don't be too hard on yourself.

2. Your baby is affected by morning sickness:

A common myth among expectant mothers is the idea that morning sickness could be harmful to their unborn child.

You can be confident that your unborn child won't be harmed by your pregnancy's nausea or vomiting.

Indeed, it may be a comforting indication that your pregnancy hormones are functioning and safeguarding your unborn child.

Morning sickness strikes mothers occasionally, but most babies are born healthy and robust.

To make sure you and your child are as comfortable as possible, it's crucial to manage your symptoms.

See your healthcare provider if you're experiencing difficulties swallowing food or staying hydrated.

They can offer advice and, if needed, recommend safe medications for you and your child.

3. Only the first trimester is associated with morning sickness:

Many people think that the occurrence of morning sickness is limited to the first trimester of pregnancy.

Although morning sickness is more common during this time of pregnancy, it can last the entire duration of your pregnancy.

Some expectant mothers still feel sick to their stomachs and throw up well into the second or even third trimester.

This prolonged period can be stressful for a pregnant woman.

Because every pregnancy is different, some mothers may find that their morning sickness subsides after the first trimester, while others may have to deal with these symptoms for longer.

Seeking support from your partner, family, or friends can help you manage morning sickness during pregnancy.

Accepting assistance can help you get through this difficult period more easily.

You don't have to do it alone.
Everyone experiences the same morning sickness.

Even though morning sickness is a typical pregnancy symptom, each pregnant woman's experience with it is very different.

Certain expectant mothers may encounter mild nausea that doesn't substantially disrupt their

everyday routines, whereas others may experience severe vomiting necessitating medical attention.

Do not hesitate to contact your healthcare provider if your morning sickness becomes especially severe.

Treatments and medications are available to help control your symptoms and protect your unborn child.

4. The cause of morning sickness is psychological:

Pregnant women often believe that morning sickness is solely psychological and that they can control it with willpower.

In actuality, pregnancy-related hormonal changes in your body are the main cause of morning sickness.

Although psychological variables may impact the intensity of symptoms, it's critical to understand that willpower is not a factor.

Be gentle with yourself and, if necessary, seek out help from family, friends, and medical professionals.

Ways to Help with Vomiting and Nausea During Pregnancy

It can be difficult to deal with morning sickness when pregnant, but there are lots of strategies to get through these symptoms and feel like you can handle it any day.

You might want to incorporate the following tactics into your everyday routine:

1. Select Boring, Easily Digestible Foods: Often known as the BRAT diet, this involves choosing foods that are bland and simple to digest, such as toast, crackers, plain rice, bananas, and applesauce.

These foods are easy on the stomach and can provide some relief from nausea.

2. Remain Hydrated: Hypoxia can exacerbate queasiness.

Drink clear liquids to stay hydrated, such as water, ginger tea, or clear juices.

If you have been vomiting, electrolyte-rich drinks can help replenish; just watch out for ingredients you don't recognize and excessive sugar.

If drinking liquids is difficult for you, you can also try sucking on ice chips.

3. Ginger: Ginger contains inherent anti-nausea qualities. Ginger supplements, tea, and candies are all options.

Some women find relief from eating fresh ginger or drinking ginger ale (be sure the beverage contains real ginger).

For support while you're on the go, you can also try Stomach Settle drops.

Ginger, mint, vitamin B6, and lemon are included in them to help ease the symptoms of sporadic nausea and morning sickness.

4. Fresh air: For some women, taking quick walks or getting outside in the fresh air helps reduce nausea.

Steer clear of hot spots and prolonged exposure to direct sunlight.

5. Sleep: Make sure you are getting adequate sleep and rest.
Anxiety can exacerbate nausea.

If you can, try to refuel during the day with quick naps.

6. **Remain Cool**: Maintain a cool, well-ventilated environment.

Nausea can occasionally worsen in hot weather.

7. **Aromatherapy**: Aromatherapy helps women feel better.

Aromas like lavender, lemon, or peppermint may help reduce nausea.

For this, scented candles or essential oils work well.

8. **Control Stress**: Relaxation methods like deep breathing, meditation, or prenatal yoga can help lower stress levels, which can help prevent nausea.

9. **Remain Upbeat**: Recall that morning sickness is a passing feeling that usually gets better as the pregnancy goes on.

Remain upbeat and concentrate on how happy you are about being pregnant.

If you experience severe or persistent morning sickness or find it difficult to keep food or liquids down, it's important to speak with your healthcare provider.

To make you feel more comfortable during this stage of your pregnancy, they can offer you individualized advice and, if required, prescription drugs.

You may come across several myths and misconceptions as an expectant mother experiencing nausea and vomiting during pregnancy.

It's critical to keep In mind that morning sickness is a typical, generally benign pregnancy symptom that differs among mothers.

While taking care of your infant, your main priority should be to maintain maximum comfort and health.

Seek assistance during this difficult time from your family, friends, and healthcare provider.

To help you manage your symptoms and make the most of this priceless time with your child, keep in mind that you're not alone and that there are resources and treatments available.

You can confidently and joyfully embrace the beauty of motherhood by dispelling these myths and putting your health first.

Chapter 2

Coping Strategies for Managing Symptoms

Sure!

Pregnancy sickness symptoms can be managed with the help of these coping mechanisms:

1. Small, Regular Meals: Throughout

the day, aim for smaller, more frequent meals rather than larger ones.

This can assist in avoiding the sensation of being overly full or empty in your stomach, which can cause nausea.

2. Keep Yourself Hydrated: It's

important to keep yourself hydrated because dehydration can make nausea worse.

Drink ginger ale, herbal teas, or water to stay hydrated throughout the day.

3. Ginger: Ginger naturally relieves nausea.

If you're feeling queasy, consider trying ginger tea, ginger candies, or ginger pills.

4. Acupressure Bands: Some women find that wearing acupressure bands on their wrists helps with nausea.

Certain wrist spots are compressed by these bands, which is said to lessen nausea.

5. Eat Less: Recognize which foods or odors make you sick, and try to stay away from them.

Dishes with strong flavors, oily or spicy dishes, and strong scents are common triggers.

6. Snack Before Bed: A lot of ladies

discover that eating a small snack before bed helps them not feel nauseous in the morning.

Select a light food that can be consumed quickly, such as toast or crackers.

7. Take Prenatal Vitamins with

Food: Taking prenatal vitamins on an empty

stomach can sometimes make nausea worse.

For the least amount of disco, try taking these with a meal or snack.

8. Relaxation: Stress and exhaustion can make nausea worse.

Prioritize getting enough sleep, and think about including deep breathing, meditation, or prenatal yoga in your daily routine as ways to decompress.

9. Cold Foods: For some women, eating something cold or frozen is more bearable than anything hot or warm.

Try cool treats such as popsicles, smoothies, or chilled fruit to see if these can ease your nausea.

10. Medication: Discuss safe medication alternatives with your healthcare provider for controlling pregnancy sickness if your nausea is severe and interfering with your ability to function.

When pregnant, nausea and vomiting can be lessened with several over-the-counter and prescription drugs.

It may take some trial and error to find the coping mechanisms that work best for you because every woman's experience with pregnancy sickness is different.

If you're having trouble controlling your symptoms, have patience with yourself, and don't be afraid to ask for help from your doctor or a support group.

You need to be among helpful people throughout this period to maintain your well-being.

This can improve physical health, reduce stress, depression, and anxiety, and lessen the likelihood of difficult pregnancies and deliveries.

The encouragement and resolve you have to make healthy lifestyle choices could also come from the people in your life.

The emotional comfort and reassurance that come with feeling well-supported can help handle fears and concerns connected to pregnancy.

Among these advantages may be a feeling of connection and belonging.

When trying to adjust to your changing body, it might help to be around people who have experienced similar changes since they can offer advice on how to manage the mental and physical changes.

What kind of social assistance is there when a woman is pregnant?

Individual differences may exist in social support.

For various people, receiving support might mean different things.

For instance, some people find that having frequent conversations with a loved one helps them feel supported, while others might require more practical support, like help with childcare or having someone prepare supper when they're feeling low.

Other people are likewise supportive.

It may be offered by pregnancy support groups, medical professionals such as midwives, doctors, or

doulas, as well as by family, friends, and other expectant mothers.

Cultural differences may also show up in the way family and friends assist you or in the kind of help you think you need.

Inadequate social connections Regretfully, many expectant mothers and new mothers feel that they aren't getting the help they need.

You may feel isolated and as though no one understands what you're going through if you're the only pregnant person in your social group or if you don't know many other new parents.

Not being in a supportive relationship or not having your family's support can also make loneliness and anxiety worse.

Women from lower-class backgrounds and members of specific ethnic minorities typically believe they receive less social help.

Because pregnancy is such a unique event, it may be especially vital to have meaningful connections and to share the experience with others.

Speak up

I know it sounds simple, yet we frequently forget to let people know what we need from them.

We may not always tell our loved ones when we're having difficulties, leading them to believe we'll let they know if we need them or that we'd rather not be bothered.

Pick up the phone or send them a text if you're feeling overwhelmed, and let them know you need a

little help, even if it just means getting together for a cup of tea and a conversation.

Never forget that assistance is there if you need it.

One crucial aspect of taking care of oneself is asking your loved ones for assistance.

Participate in prenatal groups

Joining programs and groups dedicated to pregnancy is great for meeting other pregnant people and women.

Pregnancy support groups are widely available for free; some are offered in-person, while others are offered online.

Some of them concentrate on offering emotional and practical support throughout your pregnancy, while

others are more concerned with developing social spaces for expectant mothers.

It all depends on the kind of assistance you're looking for.

Pregnancy fitness courses are also offered at neighborhood record centers and private studios, and they're a terrific opportunity to meet new people.

Attempt something novel.

By engaging in more of your favorite activities, you can also meet new individuals.

Whether it's signing up for a reading club, taking an art or language lesson, or giving your time to a worthy course.

One surefire strategy to meet someone you know you'll get along with is to connect with those who share your interests.

You never know who you might meet or what sort of assistance they might be able to provide, even if these activities are not pregnancy-focused.

Seek individual assistance

You might want to think about hiring a doula if you can afford to have one during your pregnancy.

Doulas are independent professionals who provide one-on-one care to women and individuals giving birth, providing counsel, advocacy, and both practical and emotional support during the whole pregnancy process.

Having a doula by your side to help you through your pregnancy and answer any questions you may have can be comforting and a great source of support.

Although some doulas choose to volunteer or work for the NHS, most doulas operate independently. Making connections with other mothers.

A great way to get support when pregnant is to join a mom–mom community

Get advice on managing this amazing journey, exchange experiences, and connect with other soon-to-be mothers.

During this transformative period, collective wisdom and companionship, whether through virtual events, local meetups, or online forums, can help you feel understood and supported.

Accept the experiences that other mothers who have traveled this same route have to offer, and together, enjoy the blessings and overcome the difficulties of pregnancy.

Chapter 3

Dietary Advice for Nausea

Because of shifting hormones during the first three months of pregnancy, nausea and vomiting are very prevalent.

Here are some recommendations to help with these symptoms:

1. When the stomach is empty, the symptoms feel more severe.

The nausea can be minimized by eating often (every one and a half to two hours) in modest quantities.

2. Keep drinks and solid food separate.

After consuming a drink, wait at least half an hour before eating.

The most flavored foods are those high in carbohydrates.

3. Foods that are hot, high in fat, or gassy are not well tolerated.

4. There is typically too much acid in citrus fruits and beverages.

5. Vitamins are necessary: Prenatal vitamins, if tolerated, are to be taken every day with substantial meals.

6. A daily dose of 0.4–1 mg of folic acid is advised: You can take this on its own or with the prenatal vitamins.

If you are unable to accept other vitamins, you can take Centrum or two children's chewable vitamins every day.

Two times a day, 50–100 mg of vitamin B-6 or 25 mg of vitamin B-6 are recommended to reduce nausea (must be taken twice daily).

You can buy motion sickness or sea sickness bands at pharmacies and dive shops.

7. In case you wake up throughout the night or in the morning, keep dry food of some kind close to your bed.

8. Have some lemon drops, mints, and ginger-based foods and beverages (ginger ale, ginger snaps, etc.).

Recognizing the value of a balanced diet when expecting/Dietary habit during pregnancy

The mother's and the child's health depend on being ill.
It preserves vital nutrients, promotes healthy fetal growth, and upholds the mother's well-being.

As long as the body gets the vitamins and minerals it needs, a healthy diet can help reduce the sensation of nausea.

For the best possible pregnancy experience, speaking with a healthcare provider for tailored advice is essential.

During pregnancy, you require more of several nutrients (such as iron, iodine, and folate).

The vitamins and minerals our bodies require each day are usually supplied by a diversified diet that contains the appropriate quantity of healthful foods from the five food groups.

On the other hand, pregnant women might need to take supplements of certain vitamins and minerals (such as vitamin D and folate).

Before using any supplements, speak with your physician.

To determine whether you need to take a supplement, they might advise you to do a blood test or consult a dietician.

Except in cases where a blood test has confirmed a vitamin D deficiency, you shouldn't need to take a supplement.

Pregnancy-related healthy weight gain

For the sake of both your and your unborn child's health, a steady weight gain is normal during pregnancy.

Not gaining too much weight is crucial, though. A woman who gains too much weight during her pregnancy may be more susceptible to high blood pressure and gestational diabetes, among other health problems.

Regaining too much weight might also make it challenging to drop pounds after giving birth.

An excellent strategy if you're expecting is to eat until you're satisfied and keep an eye on your weight.

Your GP, obstetrician, dietitian, or midwife can offer you advice on how to keep an eye on your weight.

This is not the time to start dieting or trying to lose weight if you are overweight during pregnancy.

Maintaining a healthy weight gain throughout pregnancy requires doing the following:

• Make wholesome meal choices from the five food groups.

• Cut back on indulgent meals and beverages that are heavy in added sugars, salt, and saturated fat (such as cakes, biscuits, and sugary drinks).

• Incorporate exercise into your pregnancy.

Consuming a healthy diet while pregnant.

There is strong evidence that the food you consume during pregnancy not only influences the development of your unborn child but also your health and well-being.

Additionally, there may be long-term effects on your child's health and well-being once they grow up.

To ensure that your baby's nutritional needs are satisfied and to promote their growth and health, make a wide variety of nutritious food choices from the five food groups.

There's no need to "eat for two," but you might find that you need to consume more of some meals to get essential nutrients.

Items to put on your pregnancy diet:

1. An assortment of variously colored and shaped fruits and vegetables.

2. Aim for two servings of fruit and five servings of veggies each day.

3. Up your daily consumption of grains and cereal foods to eight and a half servings.

4. Make largely wholegrain and high-fiber food choices.

5. Make iron-rich meal choices, like tofu or lean red meat.

For expectant mothers, diets high in iron are essential.

It is advised to have 3½ servings of meat or meat substitutes.

6. Establish a routine of consuming milk, hard cheese, yogurt, or substitutes high in calcium.

The best types are the lower-fat ones.
It is suggested to have 2.5 servings each day.

7. Drink lots of water.

8. Consume very limited amounts of meals and beverages that are heavy in added sugar, saturated fat, and salt.

Pregnancy and iron

During pregnancy, iron plays a crucial role in supporting both the mother's and the baby's health.

Here's why iron is important during pregnancy and how to ensure you're getting enough:

1. Red Blood Cell Production: Iron is essential for the production of hemoglobin, a protein in red blood cells that carries oxygen from the lungs to the rest of the body.

During pregnancy, your body produces more blood to support the growing fetus, increasing the need for iron.

2. Prevention of Anemia: Iron deficiency anemia is common during pregnancy and can lead to fatigue, weakness, and other complications.

Adequate iron intake helps prevent anemia and ensures optimal oxygen delivery for both you and your baby.

3. Fetal Development: Iron is necessary for the development of your baby's brain and overall growth.

Insufficient iron intake during pregnancy can lead to low birth weight and other developmental issues.

To ensure you're getting enough iron during pregnancy:

1. Eat Iron-Rich Foods: Include a variety of iron-rich foods in your diet, such as lean meats, poultry, fish, eggs, beans, lentils, tofu, nuts, seeds, and fortified cereals

2. Pair Iron with Vitamin C: Consuming foods rich in vitamin C, such as citrus fruits, strawberries, bell

peppers, and tomatoes, can enhance iron absorption.

Consider pairing iron-rich foods with sources of vitamin C to maximize absorption.

3 Cook in Cast Iron Cookware: Cooking acidic foods, such as tomato sauce or chili, in cast iron cookware can increase the iron content of the food.

4. Limit Iron Blockers: Some substances can inhibit iron absorption, such as calcium, caffeine, and tannins found in tea and coffee.

Try to avoid consuming these substances with iron-rich meals

5. Consider Iron Supplements: If you're unable to meet your iron needs through diet alone or if you're

At risk of iron deficiency anemia, your healthcare provider may recommend iron supplements.

It's important to take iron supplements as directed and not exceed the recommended dosage, as excessive iron intake can be harmful.

6. Regular prenatal check-ups: Your healthcare provider will monitor your iron levels throughout pregnancy and may recommend additional testing if there are concerns about iron deficiency or anemia.

Follow their guidance and discuss any questions or concerns you have about iron intake and supplementation.

Ensuring adequate iron intake during pregnancy is vital for both maternal and fetal health.

By incorporating iron-rich foods into your diet and following your healthcare provider's

recommendations, you can support a healthy pregnancy and optimal fetal development.

Iodine and gestation

Iodine is another essential nutrient during pregnancy, as it plays a critical role in fetal brain development and thyroid function.

Here's why iodine is important during gestation and how to ensure you're getting enough:

1. Brain Development: Iodine is necessary for the production of thyroid hormones, particularly thyroxine (T4) and triiodothyronine (T3).

These hormones are crucial for fetal brain development, especially during the first trimester, when the baby's brain is rapidly developing.

2. Thyroid Function: During pregnancy, the mother's thyroid gland increases hormone production to support the growing fetus.

Adequate iodine intake is essential for maintaining thyroid function and preventing thyroid disorders, such as hypothyroidism or goiter, which can negatively impact both maternal and fetal health.

To ensure you're getting enough iodine during pregnancy:

1. Consume Iodine-Rich Foods: Include iodine-rich foods in your diet, such as iodized salt, seafood (e.g., fish, shrimp, seaweed), dairy products, eggs, and fortified foods.

Iodized salt is the most common dietary source of iodine in many countries.

2. Consider Prenatal Supplements: Many prenatal vitamins contain iodine to ensure pregnant women meet their daily requirements.

If your prenatal vitamin does not contain iodine, or if you have concerns about your iodine intake, talk to your healthcare provider about taking an iodine supplement.

3. Limit Goitrogens: Some foods contain compounds called goitrogens, which can interfere with iodine uptake and thyroid function.

Examples include cruciferous vegetables (e.g. cabbage, broccoli, and cauliflower) and soy-based products.

While these foods can be part of a healthy diet, consume them in moderation and ensure you're getting enough iodine from other sources.

4. Avoid Excessive Iodine Intake: While iodine deficiency is a concern, excessive iodine intake can also be harmful, especially during pregnancy.

Avoid taking high-dose iodine supplements unless recommended by your healthcare provider, as they can disrupt thyroid function and potentially harm the developing fetus.

5. Regular prenatal check-ups: Your healthcare provider will monitor your thyroid function during

pregnancy, including thyroid hormone levels and iodine status.

If there are concerns about iodine deficiency or thyroid disorders, they may recommend additional testing or interventions.

Ensuring adequate iodine intake during pregnancy is essential for supporting fetal brain development and thyroid function.

By incorporating iodine-rich foods into your diet and following your healthcare provider's recommendations, you can help promote a healthy pregnancy and optimal fetal growth and development.

Vitamin D

Vitamin D plays a crucial role in gestation as it helps regulate calcium and phosphorus levels, which are essential for the development of the fetal skeleton and teeth.

Adequate vitamin D levels during pregnancy are important for the health of both the mother and the baby.

Pregnant women are often advised to ensure they are getting enough vitamin D through diet, sunlight

exposure, and supplementation if necessary, under the guidance of a healthcare provider.

Deficiency in vitamin D during pregnancy can lead to complications such as preeclampsia, gestational diabetes, and impaired fetal skeletal development.

Vitamin D sensitivity in expectant mothers

- A diet low in foods high in vitamin D.

- Women with certain medical conditions like obesity or diseases of the liver or kidneys that can affect vitamin D metabolism.

- Women with limited sun exposure.

- Women with darker skin tones (which require more sun exposure to produce vitamin D).

- Women who cover their skin for cultural or religious reasons.

- pregnant women with malabsorption disorders are all at risk for vitamin D deficiency.

If vitamin D supplementation is required, pregnant women should talk to their healthcare professional about their current vitamin D status.

Foods high In vitamin D

Healthy foods high in vitamin D include:

1. Egg yolks

2. Fish liver oils

3. Fortified dairy products (milk, yogurt, cheese)

4. Fortified plant-based milk (soy, almond, or oat milk)

5. Fortified cereals

6. Fortified orange juice.

Fatty fish such as salmon, tuna, and mackerel are also rich sources of vitamin D.

Furthermore, certain mushrooms that are grown in sunshine or other UV light can supply trace levels of vitamin D.

Fish mercury

Pregnant women are advised to consume two to three servings of fish each week to support both their own and the developing baby's health.

However, ladies who are currently pregnant or who plan to get pregnant in the following six months should exercise caution when choosing their seafood.

High concentrations of mercury found in certain fish species can be hazardous to a developing fetus.

Pregnant women should choose seafood based on:

- **Limit one serving (150 g) of billfish (swordfish:** Broadbill, and marlin) and shark (flake) each fortnight. During that period, no more fish may be consumed.

Or

- **No more than one serving (150 g) every week:** With no other fish consumed that week, it was roughly orange (deep sea perch) or catfish.

Or

Of any other seafood or fish (tuna, salmon, etc.).
Keep in mind that 150 g is roughly equal to two parts
of frozen, crumbed fish.

If you have occasionally eaten seafood that has a
high mercury content, don't worry.

Only when that kind of fish is consistently consumed
could there be a risk of mercury buildup in the
mother's blood?

A clean diet lowers the chance of infection.
To lower the risk of contracting listeria and
salmonella, practice good food hygiene.

Some recommendations are as follows:

• Consistently wash your hands both before and
after handling food.

- Maintain spotless kitchen surfaces.

- Keep cooked food apart from uncooked food.

- Before consuming, wash the salad, fruit, and veggies.

- Fully prepare food.

- Keep animals off of kitchen surfaces.

- When gardening or working with cat litter pans, put on rubber gloves.

- Maintain proper food storage temperatures.

Knowing what foods to avoid to reduce pregnancy nausea

It's beneficial to concentrate on bland, easily digested foods to reduce nausea during pregnancy.

Crackers, toast, dry cereal, pretzels, plain rice, plain spaghetti, applesauce, bananas, plain yogurt, broth-based soups, ginger tea or ginger ale, and short, frequent meals or snacks as opposed to large ones are a few alternatives.

Drinking enough fluids, such as water, herbal teas, or electrolyte-containing drinks, is also crucial for staying hydrated.

1. staying hydrated

Reducing your intake of oily, spicy, or overpowering foods can also help ease nausea.

For individualized dietary guidance and possible supplementation, speaking with a healthcare professional can also be helpful.

Kinds of transparent drinks

Water, sports drinks, soda water, iced tea, clear juices, coconut water, and oral rehydration treatments are the best beverages for staying hydrated and preventing nausea.

Drinks with a lot of sugar, caffeine, or dairy should be avoided, as they may exacerbate your nausea.

Furthermore, consult your physician before including any of these or other beverages regularly in your diet.

2. Crackers, bread, and pretzels

Foods that are simple, bland, and dry, such as cereal, toast, and pretzels, can soothe an upset stomach.

For this reason, they are frequently advised to those who are experiencing nausea.

3. Simple carbs' functions

These meals' starchy texture may lessen nausea symptoms by absorbing stomach acids.
Advice on how to eat these things

Store them beside your bed for a fast snack before you get up, or put a few small servings in your bag for easy access when you're on the go.

4. Cold meals

Because of their cool temperature and faint odor, cold foods like yogurt, ice cream, custard, ice pops, and chilled fruits are generally easier to handle when you're feeling queasy.

Benefits of cold or overheated food

The scents of hot foods are frequently stronger and can cause nausea, whereas the limited smell and cooling properties of cold foods can help alleviate nausea.

Examples of things to eat that are cold

Smoothies, fruit salads, blended fruit juices, and yogurt parfaits are a few of the best options for cold foods that combat nausea.

5. Soups, broths and other warm beverages

These can replenish electrolytes lost via vomiting. Help you stay hydrated and ease upset stomachs.

Advantages of broth consumption

A careful introduction to solid foods again could be through broths.

Dehydration is lessened by them.

Additionally, they provide a gentle, comforting choice in case you're feeling queasy.

Kinds of broth

Consider trying miso soup, chicken broth, or veggie broth.

These meals are nourishing and soothing choices if you're feeling queasy and unable to keep anything firm in your stomach.

6. Bananas

If you're feeling queasy, you may have a snack of bananas.

They are easy on the stomach and could aid in replenishing potassium lost due to diarrhea or vomiting.

Banana nutrients that are beneficial for nausea Vitamin B6, 27 grams of carbohydrates, 9% of the daily potassium requirement, and 105 calories are included in one medium-sized banana.

This makes it a potentially well-rounded food that can help with both nausea and energy.

How should a diet consist of bananas?

Bananas can be added to smoothies, blended with peanut butter for a quick energy boost, or eaten plain with toast or cereal for added nutrition.

7. Applesauce

This nutritious snack, along with ginger and crackers may also help reduce nausea.
Those with sensitive stomachs might find this to be an excellent option.

Using applesauce to treat nausea

Vitamins and carbs are both abundant in applesauce.

It does not hurt your stomach.

It has pectin as well.

To monitor the symptoms of diarrhea, this dietary fiber might be helpful.

Methods for Eating Applesauce

Savor some simple applesauce.
Or use it as a topping for toast or oatmeal in the morning, or combine it with cottage cheese for an extra protein boost.

A. Plain, starchy foods such as rice, potatoes, and noodles can provide some relief from nausea.

They are gentle on the stomach and provide you with the necessary calories to stay full.

The benefit of bland diets for preventing sickness

- Foods that are bland, colorless, and odorless may help you feel less queasy than those that have strong flavors.

- Simple carbs include rice, potatoes, and noodles.

They might be useful in calming troubled stomachs.

How should these foods be prepared and consumed?

Boil rice or pasta and serve either way, or opt for mashed, steamed, or boiled potatoes with mild spice.

Be certain that the food you eat is cooked simply, with few or no harsh aromas or scents.

B. Meals high in protein may provide greater relief from nausea than meals high in fat or carbohydrates, according to research.

This could be a result of proteins' role in boosting gastrin release.

The value of protein when expecting

Both the growth of your unborn child and the maintenance of your body's strength depend on protein.

It may help restore poor nutrition; therefore, it's very useful for those who are constantly sick.

Foods high in protein that can alleviate nausea

Pick lean proteins with simple seasonings or a light broth, such as grilled chicken, tofu, beans, or lentils. They provide extra nutrition without aggravating queasiness.

Herbal teas

Although there is little evidence to support their efficacy, a warm cup of herbal tea may help reduce nausea.

A cup of hot tea can also help calm an upset stomach and give you essential fluids.

Varieties of herbal drinks that help alleviate nausea

peppermint and chamomile tea, but there may be additional advantages to beverages steeped in ginger or lemon.

Advice on drinking herbal teas

Drink your tea slowly.
To prevent disturbing your stomach, take tiny sips.

For extra taste and perhaps nausea relief, experiment with different herbal concoctions or squeeze in a lemon slice.

Do not forget to consult your doctor before implementing any of the aforementioned suggestions.

Maintaining nutritional balance to assist your growing child and yourself

Getting the vitamins and minerals you require to support both your body and the developing fetus is imperative throughout pregnancy.

A balanced diet Is the key to supporting both you and your unborn child during pregnancy.

A range of foods high in important nutrients, such as calcium, iron, folate, and omega-3 fatty acids, should be included.

Choose dairy, whole grains, fruits, veggies, and lean proteins.

As recommended by your healthcare professional, drink plenty of water and think about taking prenatal vitamins.

For a healthy pregnancy, give nutrient-dense foods top priority.

Important foods for an expectant mother and her unborn child include the following:

1. Folate: The development of the fetal neural tube depends on folate, which is present in leafy greens, beans, and fortified grains.

2. Iron: Lean meats, lentils, and iron-fortified cereals are good sources of iron, which supports increased blood volume.

3. Calcium: Dairy products, leafy greens, and fortified foods are rich sources of this mineral, which is necessary for bone formation.

4. Omega-3 fatty acids: Are present in walnuts, flaxseeds, and fatty acids.

They are essential for the development of the fetus's brain and eyes.

5. Protein: essential for tissue growth; foods high in protein include dairy, eggs, lean meats, and plant-based sources.

6. Vitamin D: promotes calcium absorption; obtain it through sunshine, fortified meals, or supplements as needed.

7. Iodine: contains iodized salt, dairy products, and shellfish; supports thyroid function.

8. Vitamin C: contains citrus fruits, berries, and bell peppers; improves the absorption of iron.

For individualized advice on nutrient consumption during pregnancy, speak with your healthcare professional.

Chapter 4

A comprehensive Inventory of Medications Licensed for the Treatment of Pregnancy Sickness

Non-pharmacological approaches are often used in the first treatment of pregnancy sickness.

However, under extreme circumstances, pharmaceuticals may be considered with a physician's advice.

However, approved options consist of:

1. Pyridoxine or vitamin B6: Is a water-soluble vitamin that is often recommended for mild nausea.

2. Doxylamine: When used with vitamin B6, this antihistamine is regarded as safe for managing nausea and vomiting during pregnancy.

3. Promethazine: A prescription for an antihistamine may be issued in more serious circumstances.

4. Ondansetron: this medication is occasionally used to treat severe nausea and vomiting; its safety during pregnancy is currently being studied.

It's crucial to see a medical expert before taking this drug.

Consult your doctor to ensure that any medications you take while pregnant are safe and appropriate for your unique situation before beginning.

Before undergoing any medical procedure, one should always weigh the benefits and drawbacks.

Consult a healthcare provider to find out more about:

Advantages:

Symptom relief: Interventions can alleviate pain or treat illnesses.

Fetal Health: Sometimes interventions can improve the baby's surroundings.

Risks:

Side effects: Medication or treatment side effects might affect both the mother and the fetus.

Unknown Long-Term Effects: It may be challenging to forecast the effects of some therapies due to a lack of long-term data.

Potential Impact on Pregnancy: Certain operations may carry risks for the developing fetus.

Your healthcare provider will provide you with tailored advice based on your health, the specific intervention, and our current understanding of its implications during pregnancy.

Making decisions requires open channels of communication.

Pregnant women may require medication to treat new or pre-existing health conditions.

Additionally, taking specific vitamins is advised while pregnant.

A pregnant woman should see a doctor before using any medication, including over-the-counter drugs, or dietary supplements, including medicinal plants.

If at all possible, women who are taking medication and intend to get pregnant should see a doctor before getting pregnant to see whether or not their existing prescriptions need to be modified or stopped. (See also Medicine and Pregnancy at the Centers for Disease Control and Prevention.)

Certain drugs have side effects even after they are stopped because they remain in the body.

For instance, the drug isotretinoin, which treats skin conditions, is kept in fat beneath the skin and delivered gradually over weeks.

If a woman falls pregnant within two weeks of stopping isotretinoin, birth abnormalities may result.

It is therefore recommended that women delay getting pregnant for at least three to four weeks following the cessation of treatment.

Depending on what is presently known about a drug's safety during pregnancy, government organizations that regulate drug safety may categorize certain medications.

Research on side effects reported by patients taking the medicine, as well as research on humans and animals.

Pregnant women are often advised by doctors to take medications based on the research that is currently available, the medication's value to the pregnant woman's health, and the availability of alternative treatments that pose less risk to the woman and fetus.

Pregnant women may get medication if the advantages outweigh the hazards.

Pregnant women are advised to have this

vaccination since it is safe to administer during pregnancy.

1. Pregnant women who will become pregnant or who are pregnant during flu season should consider getting the influenza (flu) vaccine.

2. Whenever possible, tetanus, diphtheria, and pertussis (Tdap) vaccines should be given in the third trimester to protect against whooping cough, often known as pertussis.

3. COVID-19 vaccination: This is for those who are nursing, trying to get pregnant, pregnant right now, or who may get pregnant in the future.

There is growing evidence that this COVID-19 vaccination given during pregnancy is safe and effective.

These results indicate that the benefits of receiving the COVID-19 vaccine before becoming pregnant outweigh any potential or known risks related to vaccination.

Refer to FDA Approves First Vaccine to Prevent RSV in Infants While Pregnant.

The United States Food and Drug Administration (FDA) approved the use of the respiratory syncytial virus (RSV) vaccination in pregnant women between 32 and 36 weeks, along with the use of the vaccine in August 2023.

The FDA did, however, advise against administering the vaccine before 32 weeks of pregnancy.

Some issues that may affect the fetus are renal damage, growth limitation, or inadequate growth before birth, among other conditions.

Pregnant women are also not prescribed spironolactone.

This medication may induce the development of feminine traits in a male fetus; this process is referred to as "feminization.

Digoxin penetrates the placenta quickly and is used to treat heart failure and some abnormal heart rhythms.

However, digoxin usually has minimal effects on the newborn before or after delivery when taken as directed.

Antidepressant Use During Pregnancy

Pregnant women are often prescribed antidepressants, particularly selective serotonin reuptake inhibitors (SSRIs) such as sertraline, due to the high prevalence of clinical depression during this time.

For expecting moms, the advantages of treating depression usually outweigh the risks. Paroxetine appears to raise the chance of congenital cardiac abnormalities.

Consequently, if a pregnant woman takes paroxetine, echocardiography should be done to evaluate the fetus's heart.

However, this danger is not increased by other SSRIs.

Using antidepressants while pregnant raises the baby's risk of experiencing withdrawal symptoms, such as agitation and shaking.

To prevent these side effects, doctors may gradually reduce the dosage of antidepressants during the third trimester and cease the medicine before the baby is born.

Nevertheless, if a woman has severe depressive symptoms or if a lower dosage makes her symptoms worse, antidepressants should be taken.

Pregnancy depression can progress to postpartum depression, which requires therapy and entails a major mood shift.

Antiviral medications during pregnancy

Antiviral drugs (such as ritonavir and zidovudine for HIV infection) have been safely used during pregnancy for a long time.

Certain antiviral drugs, however, may pose risks to the growing fetus.

For example, some data suggests that some HIV regimens involving a mix of antiviral drugs may raise

the frequency of cleft lip and palate during the first trimester.

When treating a pregnant patient with early mild to moderate COVID-19, the treatment team may consider the advantages and disadvantages of using remdesivir vs. nirmatrelvir-ritonavir.

When considering the use of baricitinib or tocilizumab, pregnant patients hospitalized with COVID-19 may also be evaluated.

The majority of medical professionals agree that theoretical worries regarding the safety of antiviral drugs shouldn't stop pregnant women from using them.

Since treatment for influenza is most effective when administered within 48 hours of the onset of symptoms, pregnant women who get the illness should seek treatment as soon as possible.

However, treatment lowers the risk of serious consequences at any stage of the disease.
There aren't any well-designed studies on zanamivir and oseltamivir in expectant mothers.

However, several observational studies indicate that using zanamivir or oseltamivir while pregnant does not raise the risk of side effects.

It Is advised that all expectant mothers who are or will become pregnant during flu season receive the vaccination against influenza.

Using acyclovir topically or orally to treat the herpes simplex virus appears to be safe during pregnancy.

Consulting with healthcare professionals to determine the best choice.

Yes, speaking with medical professionals is essential to determining the best course of action when pregnant.

They can:

1. Evaluate your health

Taking into account your past medical history, present state of health, and any particular conditions.

2. Talk about risks and benefits

Provide thorough details regarding possible interventions, including any risks involved and their effects

3. Customize suggestions

Make recommendations based on your particular requirements and situation.

4. Respond to questions and concerns

Throughout the decision-making process, respond to questions and concerns and offer assistance.

You can make decisions that are in line with your baby's health and well-being by keeping lines of communication open and transparent with your healthcare team.

If I'm pregnant, what are my options?

Choosing an unintended pregnancy is a private matter. Although having accurate information and support is helpful, only you can decide what's best for you.

Unexpected pregnancy might be unpleasant, but it's a typical occurrence—over half of all American women have been pregnant unintentionally at some point in their lives.

Pregnant women have the following three options:

1. Parenting: conceiving a child and nurturing them.

2. Abortion: taking medicine or having a medical procedure to end a pregnancy.

3. Adoption: giving birth and giving your child up to a new family or individual for life.

Sometimes it's easy to decide how to handle an unanticipated pregnancy.

At times, it can be challenging or intricate. Everybody's circumstances are unique, and your choice is highly personal.

Since you are the only one in your shoes, the choice is entirely yours.

What may I consider when making a decision?

Most people consider several factors carefully before deciding whether to have an unintended pregnancy, including their family, relationships, education, employment, finances, life goals, health, safety, and personal views.

Think about how parenting, adoption, and abortion make you feel.

What desires do you have for your future as well as the future of your family?

Posing queries to oneself such as these could be beneficial:

A. How would my choice impact my future.?

B. How would my choice impact other kids or my family?

C. Are my body and mind prepared for pregnancy and childbirth?

D. Am I now prepared to be a parent?

E. Regarding adoption, parenting, or abortion, do I have strong personal or religious convictions?

F. Am I under any pressure to choose a particular option?

G. Could my choice have unintended consequences for my life?

H. Will my partner, my family, and my friends support my choice?

There are a lot of things to take into account, and it's quite acceptable to experience a wide range of emotions while making decisions.

Many people rely on other people's encouragement and counsel while they make decisions.

It's wise to surround yourself with individuals that you know will accept you and not pass judgment.

Who can I discuss my options with?

When you're trying to decide what to do about an unwanted pregnancy, talking with your spouse, a member of your family, a friend, a trusted religious advisor, or a counselor can be beneficial.

Whatever your decision regarding your pregnancy, the compassionate staff at your neighborhood.

Planned parenthood health center is here to answer your questions, provide you with accurate,

nonjudgmental information about all of your options, and provide support while you make it.

In addition, Planned Parenthood provides prenatal care, adoption, and abortion services or can connect you with local providers of these services.

You may discuss your choice with private physicians and other family planning facilities.

When searching for a reputable health facility, use caution.

Pregnancy services are purportedly offered by certain fraudulent clinics.

These are run by individuals who oppose abortion and don't think it's appropriate to inform you of all of your pregnancy alternatives.

They go by the name of crisis pregnancy centers. To try to terrify or shame somebody into selecting an abortion, they might use manipulation and lies.

With names that are similar to those of Planned Parenthood health centers or other legitimate medical facilities, crisis pregnancy clinics frequently have locations that are close by.

Their purpose Is to mislead patients into attending their clinic instead.
Expand your knowledge of crisis pregnancy centers.

At what point must I make a choice?

It's crucial to take the time necessary to make the best choice for you.

However, the choices you have may change depending on when you make them.

To receive the best medical care available, it is wise to decide what you want to accomplish as soon as you can.

Since abortion is prohibited in some places, scheduling an appointment may take longer, and you may have to travel a distance to have one if you're thinking about getting one.

Additionally, finding a physician willing to perform an abortion after the first trimester, or the 12th week of pregnancy, may be more difficult.

Get prenatal care as soon as you can if there's a chance your pregnancy will go on, regardless of whether you decide to keep the kid or give it up for adoption.

Additionally, to ensure your health and the well-being of your unborn child, schedule prenatal appointments with your physician regularly.

At any stage of your pregnancy, if adoption is on your mind, you have the option to place your child for adoption.

After the baby is delivered, the adoption procedure might be able to begin.
How soon you decide to create an adoption plan will depend on your needs and circumstances.

The knowledgeable staff at your neighborhood Planned Parenthood health facility is available to assist and advise you.

Schedule a visit so that, regardless of your choice, you can maintain your health.

Recognizing the Value of Frequent Examinations and Surveillance

Throughout pregnancy, routine examinations and monitoring are essential for several reasons, including:

1. Fetal development

The ability to track a baby's growth and development helps healthcare professionals make sure everything is going according to plan.

2. Maternal Health

Prenatal exams help detect and treat any health problems that may develop in the mother, guaranteeing her well-being through the pregnancy.

3. Preventive care facilitates

The early identification of possible problems, enabling prompt management and action to avert more significant problems.

4. Screening for illnesses

Timely care is made possible by the identification of illnesses, including gestational diabetes and preeclampsia, through routine testing and screenings.

Personalized advice on nutrition and lifestyle to support a healthy pregnancy can be provided by healthcare experts.

5. Emotional Support

Routine examinations offer a chance to talk about any worries or emotional difficulties, guaranteeing all-encompassing care for mental and physical health.

The Advantages of Frequent Check-Ups During Pregnancy

It's crucial to attend your routine antenatal checkups for peace of mind, as pregnancy might cause worry.

You have the opportunity to ask your doctor whatever you want during these examinations, and they can make sure both you and your child are healthy.

You might feel more at rest knowing that your doctor can help you manage any other symptoms you may be experiencing during these check-ups.

The doctor can perform the required tests and assist you with birth planning during these check-ups.

In addition to learning more about breastfeeding and what to expect after birthing, you will be able to see your baby during your 3D/4D scan and ultrasound.

In general, preventive measures like routine monitoring help to ensure a safe pregnancy and quickly address any problems.

You will be offered several examinations, tests, and scans as part of your prenatal care.

In Australia, as part of standard prenatal care, some tests are provided to all women.

If there is a higher chance of complications for you or your unborn child, or if you have any concerns while you are pregnant, more testing may be recommended.

It Is entirely up to you whether or not to take any of the suggested tests.

Not all issues will be apparent before your child is born, but many will.

During prenatal care, two primary test types are provided:

1 Screening tests: These can indicate whether your kid is more likely to have a problem, but they are not able to definitively identify the issue.

2. Diagnostic testing: which provides a considerably higher degree of assurance regarding the health of your child.

Depending on whether you're giving birth at home, at a birthing center, in a public or private hospital, or someplace else in your community, your examinations and testing may be performed there.

Additionally, it could reveal if your obstetrician, midwife, or doctor performs your check-ups.

The antenatal care you select, whether you've had a previous pregnancy, and whether you're experiencing any issues may all have an impact on the time and quantity of some of the appointments and tests listed below.

The examinations, screenings, and tests that you would typically be recommended for a straightforward pregnancy are as follows

First encounter:

• Verification that you are expecting.

• determining the number of weeks you are pregnant and the approximate date of your delivery.

If the date is unclear, you might be offered an ultrasound scan.

• blood pressure, weight, and stature.

• Health and family background.

• A blood test that looks for hepatitis B, hepatitis C, syphilis, chlamydia, HIV, anemia, rubella immunity, and other conditions.

• Urine test to detect urinary tract infection or bladder infection.

• Down syndrome screening.

• Screening for cervical cancer to look for any symptoms of the disease or the human papillomavirus (HPV).

• If you are suspected of having a vitamin D deficiency, a test might be recommended.

You will typically talk with your doctor or midwife about the following during your check-up:

- The medications you now take.

- If you use alcohol or smoke,

- If you'd like to get vaccinated against influenza,

- Which dietary supplements, if any, should you take or avoid?

- The alternatives you have for prenatal care

- Where to get prenatal classes and more information.

- evaluating your health and determining whether you have any issues.

A blood glucose tolerance test is used to diagnose diabetes.

28 days

- blood pressure.

- Measuring your belly (palpating your abdomen) to determine the baby's growth.

- Evaluating your health and determining whether you have any issues.

- Monitor your infant's respiration and heart rate.

- Talking about your delivery strategy and bringing your child home.

- A blood test to determine blood platelet counts and anemia.

- An injection of anti-D immunoglobulin may be administered if your blood type is Rh-negative.

- Vaccination against pertussis.

- Urine test, if elevated blood pressure or symptoms of a urinary tract infection occur.

32-week period.

- blood pressure.

- Assessing the size of your baby by palpating your abdomen.

- Evaluating your health and determining whether you have any issues.

- Monitoring the heartbeat and motions of the urine test if elevated blood pressure or symptoms of a urinary tract infection occur.

Between 34 and 36 weeks

- Blood pressure.

- Assessing the size of your baby by palpating your abdomen.

- Evaluating your health and determining whether you have any issues.

- Monitoring the heartbeat and motions of your test if elevated blood pressure or symptoms of a urinary tract infection occur.

- Vaginal swab testing for GBS (group B streptococci).

- You might receive a second anti-D immunoglobulin injection if you have Rh-negative blood.

- Measuring the baby's presentation, or how high they are, and their station, or how far down their head has slid into your pelvis.

38 and 39 weeks

- Blood pressure.

- Assessing the size of your baby by palpating your abdomen.

- Evaluating your health and determining whether you have any issues.

- Monitor your infant's respiration and heart rate.

- If elevated blood pressure or symptoms of a urinary tract infection occur.

- Evaluating the station and display.

41-40 weeks

- Blood pressure.

- Assessing the size of your baby by palpating your abdomen.

- Evaluating your health and determining whether you have any issues.

- Monitor your infant's respiration and heart rate.

- Urine that elevated blood pressure or symptoms of a urinary tract infection occur.

- Evaluating the station and display.

- Check the baby's heartbeat and the amount of fluid surrounding them if you haven't given birth yet.

- In addition to the examinations, scans, and testing, your GP, midwife, or obstetrician may recommend additional tests in addition to the examinations, scans, and tests mentioned above, based on your circumstances and risk factors.

These might consist of:

1. Chorionic villus sampling (CVS), in which a tiny portion of the placenta of the infant is taken to check for chromosomal abnormalities like Down syndrome.

Usually, between weeks 11 and 13, if not earlier, if a problem is suspected, this procedure is carried out.

2. Non-invasive prenatal testing (NIPT): This very accurate test can identify some additional abnormalities as well as Down syndrome.

Starting around week ten of pregnancy, it can be done.

3. A nuchal translucency scan, which examines the back of your child's neck to determine whether Down syndrome is a possibility.

This test is performed between weeks 11 and 14 of pregnancy, and it may be done concurrently with the dating ultrasound.

A tiny sample of amniotic fluid—the fluid surrounding the baby—is extracted during an amniocentesis procedure to determine whether the child has a chromosomal issue or any other anomaly.

This is often carried out at 15 to 20 weeks, or sooner if there is an issue.

Conclusion

The various facets of pregnancy sickness have been examined in this book, along with its causes, symptoms, and various treatment approaches.

The Intention has always been to arm expectant moms with information to help them through this difficult but fleeting stage, from dietary advice to possible medical procedures.

Readers can face this journey with resilience, knowledge, and confidence if they have a thorough awareness of the nuances of pregnancy.

May every reader starting on the amazing and life-changing journey of parenting find that this information makes for a healthier, more comfortable pregnancy experience.